One of Service

Michael Yanuck MD PhD

For the physicians who trained me.

And for Angie and her family.

The names of those described here have been changed and information about them hidden so to disguise their identities.

Bioenergy is a technique that can be learned and it is my hope that this book will serve as a first step in acquiring that skill.

The best way to find yourself is to lose yourself in the service of others.
~Mahatma Gandhi.

INTRODUCTION

At the Hollywood General Hospital, the Chairman of Neurology, Dr. Lowell Franklin, summoned me to his office.

"I received your letter," he said. "Are you certain that you want to leave Hollywood General?"

"Yes, sir," I said. "I've made up my mind."

"Because of the added call," he said.

I was silent.

"I've had time to look into the matter, and I agree with you completely," he responded. "You're no slacker. I know that. You've done well and you're conscientious. You've been on the ward continuously for the past six months. You've had it rough. You've been working understaffed, and admitted more patients than any other first year Resident in our program."

He edged closer.

"Let me tell you something - and this is just between you and me," he said. "What you have to understand is a lot of the people in this program are assholes, and here I'm not talking about just the Residents."

He sat back.

"But they're not willing to make exceptions," he added.

He turned to the side, then looked at me.

"You finish the program," he said, "and I'll get you any fellowship in the country. I'll put you on fast track to become an academician. If it isn't a career in research that you want, then I'll make you rich."

"I'm grateful for your training, Dr. Franklin," I responded. "You've taught me how an understanding of Neurology can save lives, and I intend to take that with me everywhere I go. But I've accepted a position at Watts General now and plan to go back there."

"Where you did your internship," he responded. His speech was slow and thoughtful. "South-Central. They need you there."

Then, he leaned back again.

"But it has a bad reputation," he continued, resuming his familiar detached tone. "You won't see interesting cases. You'll be bored intellectually. Besides, they don't have a Neurology program. What will you do?"

"I'll study Internal Medicine," I answered.

"Hmm," he said, narrowing his gaze. "If it's Internal Medicine that you want, why don't you stay here? You really think that you'll get better training at Watts General?"

As I stood considering, a vision of the warm, enlightened faces of the attending physicians I knew at Watts General entered my head. My chest expanded and the weight of my doubts lifted.

"Yes," I said. "Yes…"

CHAPTER ONE

Arriving home late at the apartment Kate met me at the door.

"I've already put the children to bed," she whispered.

I peeked into the children's room: Lori, the oldest, age nine, occupied the loft; underneath was Alyssa, Kate's youngest, age two. Adjacent was the trundle bed that held Tommy, Calvin and Ashley, ages seven, five and four.

Kate crept behind me.

"You know what happened today," she said. "Ashley was saying to Alyssa, 'Where's Mike?', just to tease her and see what she'd do. Alyssa was in her chair. Earlier in the morning we had told her that you had to go back to work. I think that she'd been watching a video. She looked around, then got up, put her head in the chair and sobbed."

Just then, Alyssa awoke and looked at me.

"Hi Mike," she chirped.

I entered the room and knelt at the bed.

"I dreamed," she continued. "I dreamed of a sand castle. It got broke. It got broke by friends."

"You want to tell your mom about your dream?" I asked. "You wait here. I'll get her."

But turning, she clung to my back and hitched a ride to her mother's room. Kate was in bed.

"Do you want to lie on mommy's tummy?" Kate asked, smiling.

"If I go on your tummy," Alyssa responded, unsure, "will it growl?"

We laughed...

3

CHAPTER TWO

Arriving at Watts General the next morning, the Internal Medicine Department Chairman, Dr. Shigura, was already standing in front of a room full of Residents discussing challenges for the year ahead. Then, seeing me, his countenance immediately brightened.

"And here's our returning 'Outstanding PGY-1 Resident'!" he announced, citing the last award I'd received just before leaving. "Dr. Michael Yanuck."

I smiled – But scanning the group I saw very few familiar faces and felt sad that so many of the Residents I'd trained with were now gone.

Walking onto the ward, a new crop of Interns were milling about the nurses station – pulling out charts and looking young but quite serious.

Brand new, full-fledged doctors, I thought, watching. On their first day.

Just then, two Interns approached me.

"Dr. Yanuck, I'm Patel," said the first. "I've been assigned to your team."

"And I'm Anthony," said the second. "I've also been assigned to you."

Attending patients Anthony was slow and methodical; Patel was observant and resourceful; both were hard working and I felt exceedingly fortunate.

Around 5PM I told Patel to go home.

"You have a lot to absorb," I said. "Anthony and I are on-call tonight, so we'll take care of the patients from here."

4

"You are a good teacher, Dr. Yanuck," he said. "All the rest of the Interns and Residents are foreign grads. You are the only one trained in an American school. You went to Midland – that's a famous place. Hollywood has a good reputation. Why would you leave there to come here?"

I sat beside him.

"There were many reasons," I said. "Mostly, I left because I felt that the program was compromising both me and my patients. When finally the problems of sleep deprivation were formally published, revealing the mistakes Residents were making as a result of being up all night, residency reforms were put in place to curtail those hours. But the Neurology Department decided it wasn't going to adopt those changes; instead, we were made to work even harder! This was because the Internal Medicine Residents rotating with Neurology were now leaving early; where we'd previously worked alongside each other, now all the work was falling to us after being up all night, putting patients at even more risk.

"Then, one of the Neurology Residents dropped out, and overnight call went from every fourth night to every third. Throughout the year I'd been praised for my willingness to take the extra call. But, when I got sick, the Department decided that I needed to be punished. Initially, the Chairman, Dr. Franklin, rescinded the punitive measures, but others in the Department applied pressure, and he relented. I didn't see things changing, so I offered my resignation.

"I was invited to join the Medicine program at Hollywood, but the way their Interns and Residents had left early while we were so overburdened soured my feeling for the Department. During my internship at Watts General that simply didn't happen - You wouldn't leave a fellow Resident who was overworked.

"That isn't to say that Watts General doesn't have its problems. But moral authority isn't one of them. In this Department, if our Chairman, Dr. Shigura, asks for my all, it's because it's absolutely needed. That's why I want to be here."

He stared down.

"Does that mean you're letting go of your dream of becoming a Neurologist?" he asked.

I subtly shook my head.

"I don't know," I said…

CHAPTER THREE

In the evening I stared out from the terrace. Kate stepped out of the apartment and moved beside me.

"Alyssa doesn't want to go for walks anymore," I confided.

"She's past that, Mike," Kate responded. "She's grown out of that stage."

I nodded.

"I can remember every walk that I ever took with Alyssa during my Internship at Watts General," I said. "The swaying of the trees in the Santa Ana winds, the lights from the beach, and Alyssa falling asleep on my shoulder. I can remember all those times as though they're etched upon my consciousness. Funny, though - I can't seem to remember a single one of them after starting at Hollywood. After that, my mind's a blur."

Kate took my hand.

"Mike, you were so depleted," she said. "They never gave you any rest."

She eyed the letter I was holding.

"Who is that from?" she asked.

"Shoniah," I responded. "Ethel's daughter. Would you like to read it?"

In the darkness she held the letter close to her face, reading intently.

Dear Mike,

I'm surprised that you are not interested in Neurology anymore. You've worked so hard to get where you are now. I'm sure you have given it a great deal of thought so perhaps you are doing the best thing for yourself.

Are you doing bioenergy? If so, are you getting some good results? I hope your health is back to normal – I trust you are okay.
Take care,
Shoniah

Pulling her hands down, Kate sighed.

"Mike, the residency at Hollywood General was making you miserable," she said. "It was taking all of us down with you."

Numb, I kept my eyes averted.

"Mike, think of what a gift it is," she pleaded. "Think about what you can give to those patients at Watts General – all of your experience and training. You have a kind of training that none of the other Residents over there has. Think of how much you can show them. You don't think that God has a design in that? When are you going to have some faith?"

Kate lowered her head, then went back inside. Staring into the night sky, my thoughts drifted to that last conversation with Dr. Arnold; calling me at home from Hollywood General; insisting I come in even when I was so dizzy with fever I could hardly sit up straight to come to the phone.

"Other people have the flu," he asserted, "and they're still working."

"If it's absolutely necessary, I'll come in," I responded.

"Yeah, I think you should be here with everybody else," he said. "Now, you're breaking up other people's schedules just because you feel sick. I mean, how would you feel if someone was making you come in just because they felt sick? I don't think that's the way to do things."

I listened, disbelieving.

"So?" he demanded. "Do you think you're too sick to come in?"

A calm settled over me.

"Dr. Arnold, I'm in no condition to work," I responded. "Patient care would be compromised."

"Okay, then," he responded. "Fine."

He hung up.

Looking out now, I dropped my head...

CHAPTER FOUR

"Dr. Yanuck, this is Patel. We have a patient that we picked up from Neurosurgery. Hey, can you take a look at him? He's having difficulty breathing."

On the ward the patient was barely conscious.

"He was alright a little while ago," said Patel. "He was breathing comfortably, and then, all of a sudden, he just stopped…"

As I entered the ward, the Neurologist, Dr. Cho, was walking in the other direction.

"Why they don't do surgery?!" he called out in frustration. "Neurosurgery no good here!"

He scoffed off the ward. I examined the patient.

"Patel, the patient's problem isn't in his lungs," I said. "It's in his brain. The respiratory centers of the brainstem are failing."

Patel had the patient's head CT. We viewed it through the light-box. The brain was swollen, with white dots scattered throughout.

"These are calcifications caused by Cysticercosis – a parasite that infects the brain," I said. "The patient needs immediate surgical intervention. Why did Neurosurgery transfer him?"

"He was newly diagnosed with HIV," he said. "After that, they said that he wasn't a surgical candidate…"

The patient became comatose, and had to be intubated. I insisted that Neurosurgery re-evaluate the patient, and a Resident with that service strut onto the unit.

"This patient is not a surgical candidate," he insisted.

"I don't understand," I said. "He's herniating right in front of us. If you don't take him to the operating room now, he'll die."

"There's no way he's going to surgery!" the Resident responded. "There's no way it's gonna happen!... Are you insisting on this of your own volition?!... Did someone instruct you to do it?!..."

CHAPTER FIVE

Dr. Shigura summoned me to his office.

"Mike, a complaint was filed against you," he said. "It came from Neurosurgery."

I nodded.

"I spoke to the others who witnessed the exchange," he continued. "Your intern, Dr. Patel, spoke very highly of you. He said that if it hadn't been for your training in Neurology, the patient wouldn't have had a chance."

He handed me an envelope marked, 'Confidential.' I read in silence.

To: Arthur Webb, MD, Chairman, Department of Neurosurgery
From: Thomas Shigura, MD, Chairman, Department of Internal Medicine
Subj: House Staff Complaint

I am responding to a written complaint by one of your Residents regarding the conduct and behavior of Dr. Michael Yanuck. I have assessed the situation on the behalf of Dr. Yanuck, and find no fault.

I believe this is the second complaint our Department has received this past week against a specific Resident by Neurosurgery. It is not as important to determine who is at fault as the unhealthy professional relationship that could escalate and ultimately jeopardize patient care. Our two Departments have traditionally worked well together in the management of the most critically ill patients in the hospital. It is essential that we have a good working relationship...

Re-placing the letter in the envelop, I returned it with a nod.

"How is it going, Mike?" Dr. Shigura asked, smiling. "Are you happy to be back here?"

I hesitated.

"I'm reapplying to Neurology programs," I said.

"Alright," he responded. "Good luck."

He went back to the mound of papers and folders at his desk...

Neurology Application – Personal Statement

It was near the end of medical school that I discovered my interest in Neurology. On the second day of my Neurology rotation I was examining a patient; he complained of back pain, but there was something peculiar about his exam; when I told my Resident, he examined the patient with me, pointing to differences in muscle bulk, changes in reflexes, and, as the exam continued, I was gripped by a feeling of excitement, like beholding a symphony, reaching its climax, as a clinical diagnosis was reached.

In addition to my medical degree, I was awarded a doctorate for my work in cancer vaccine development at the National Institutes of Health. It was during my years at the NIH that I also realized, first-hand, the limitations of medicine: I suffered a leg injury, and chronic pain significantly compromised my abilities. Although I sought help from a number of medical specialists, I received little benefit. As a last resort I turned to alternative healers, and slowly made progress in healing. I thought I might leave conventional medicine altogether, but, returning to medical school, two things happened: The first was the epiphany at the Neurology clinic. The second was a chance reunion with a friend diagnosed with pancreatic cancer, and caring for her the last months of her life I rediscovered the vital role conventional medical care, and the role I had to play in it.

I chose Watts General Hospital to do my internship because I wanted to come home to Los Angeles and work in a county setting, serving the underserved and underprivileged.

My outside activities include dance, writing and the Chinese healing art of Chi Gong...

CHAPTER SIX

At the Coolidge Medical Center I was invited to interview for a second year Neurology position. I'd enjoyed my interactions with the Residents, but when it was time to interview with the Chairman of that Department, he shook my hand as though throwing it back at me.

"I saw your personal statement," he said, frowning. "I read about your 'adventures'."

He turned his back, then sat stiffly behind his desk.

"What is 'Chi Gong'?" he asked.

"It's a Chinese healing art," I responded, collegially. "It's built on the concept that there's an universal life force that runs through all things and its practice can facilitate healing."

"How do you use it?" he said.

"By helping to remove energy imbalances from the body," I replied. "I can demonstrate it for you, if you like?"

I held out my hand.

"Feel over my hand," I offered, "and see if you don't perceive something."

He moved his hand over mine, then stopped over the center of my palm and raised his brows.

"Well, what if I do feel something?" he asked.

"Then, you've taken your first step," I said…

CHAPTER SEVEN

In the darkness beyond a doorway, my departed friend, Ethel –
her body wasted, eyes glowing red – lay calling out.
"I don't want to die," she said. "I don't want to die..."

Awakening from the dream, I drew a deep breath.
Rising from the bed I drafted a letter to my former Internal
Medicine professor at the Midland College of Medicine.

Hi Dr. Brand,
I wasn't accepted into Coolidge's Neurology program. I'll continue to
look for programs elsewhere...

CHAPTER EIGHT

On-call for admitting patients to the ward from the Emergency Department, I responded to a page.

"Dr. Yanuck, this is ER Resident, Leslie Schultz. We have a patient that we want to admit to the floor. She has a urine tox screen that's positive for amphetamines and came here altered. Would you please write the orders for her?..."

In the Emergency Room the patient sat in a gurney cradling her head in her hands.

"Are you okay?" I asked.

"I have a really bad headache," she responded.

After reviewing the chart, I went to Dr. Schultz.

"It says here that the patient has had three witnessed seizures since she's come to the ER," I commented.

"Amphetamines can produce seizures," Schultz responded.

"But three of them in the couple of hours that she's been here you can't just attribute to amphetamines alone," I explained. "We need to look for other causes. She has a stiff neck and headache - She could have meningitis."

"But she doesn't have a fever!" Schultz exclaimed in a shrill voice.

"Just because she doesn't have all the classic symptoms doesn't mean we shouldn't look it," I countered. "Every minute counts."

"She's a drug addict!" Schultz cried.

"All the more reason to look for other causes and take her complaints seriously," I said.

Schultz went to her attending, Dr. Rake. Rake gave me a stern look.

"Are you questioning my diagnosis?" he demanded. "Are you listening to me, Yanuck? Are you listening? You feel that everyone is here to play!"

"I've never had this kind of problem before with an Internal Medicine Resident," he continued. "I will write you up for this. I will report you to our Chairman..."

CHAPTER NINE

In the morning Dr. Aziz met me in the Emergency room.

"That seizing lady that you saw last night didn't make it," he said. "They did the lumbar puncture. It showed that she had meningitis. It was just like you said, but the disease had progressed too far before we could get her to the unit. She died in the Emergency room."

Speechless, I lowered my gaze.

"You did everything that you could, Mike," he said. "You couldn't have done anything more. If it had been another Medicine Resident down here, they wouldn't have stood up to the emergency room, and admitted the patient to the ward. You didn't. You should be proud."

"Do you remember during your internship, Mike?" he continued. "There was a patient with sepsis who was admitted to the ward. I was your attending then. You called me. You were upset and frightened. 'Dr. Aziz,' you said. 'The patient is bleeding, and I can't get it to stop.'"

Of course I remembered, I thought. The patient had held out his arms to me. "Help me, doctor," he'd cried. "Help me." It was an image I didn't think I'd ever forget.

"It was a complicated case," he continued. "After you called, we sent the patient to the Intensive Care Unit. Still, he died because he didn't receive treatment in time. It was too late for him."

"It was a bad mistake," he said. "I didn't tell you at the time, but the next day I went to the Medical Resident overseeing admissions from the emergency room and asked him why he had let the patient go to a regular bed when it was obvious that he needed better care? He told me that it was because the emergency room had pressured him, so he admitted the patient to the ward even though he was too sick. It was a fatal mistake, and it cost the patient his life. Tonight, you kept that from happening to another Intern, so that he would not have to experience what you did, and watch a senseless loss of life.

"Even when you were an Intern, you had a compassion for others that defied reason. I have never seen that in anyone – before or since. There is no explaining it. The answer is simply that you have been born with a gift from God. It is a blessing, but it will mark you for the rest of your life. Your patients will love you, but your peers will hate, criticize, ridicule and attack you because you possess something that they lack.

"You left Hollywood because they abused you. You wouldn't have walked away if they told you they needed you. They let you go – It's their loss, and our gain.

"I know that you have made plans to go back to Neurology, although I don't know why? Only you can answer that question – I can't. Nevertheless, it is my hope that you will finish the program here, because you're desperately needed."

"Remember, Mike," he concluded. "The artist loves his work. God does not create a person who He does not love. By caring for His creations, you honor Him..."

CHAPTER TEN

An African American man wearing faded denim overalls sat beside me at a bus stop. Looking like a hobo, I feared that he'd rob me and made to run. But my limbs were so leaden and heavy that I could barely move, and scurrying off, the hobo kept pace alongside me, laughing and good-naturedly taunting me...

Awakening, I sat up in bed.

The decision to go back to Watts General is going to ruin my career, I ruminated. It has a bad reputation. The patients aren't intellectually stimulating. I should have never left Hollywood.

Kate lay asleep beside me.

Five kids? I disparaged.

The night before, we'd argued.

"You've got to figure out what you're going to do," she'd demanded. "Are you going to finish your residency at Watts General? Are you going to look for another place to do Neurology? You've got to decide."

"It's not like you're single," she'd continued. "You've got six people who are dependent on you. You can't just keep leaving us in limbo..."

"I don't know if I can do it," I told my friend, Al Lee. "It might be too much for me."

"Mike, about a week ago I had a revelation," he said. "'The most important thing in life is to give and receive unconditional love.' That's what it told me..."

Sitting by the door a bright white light shined into the room.

"Open your clinic," a voice in my head said...

Kate appeared, smiling.

"I just wanted to tell you before I forgot," Kate said. "Alyssa and I were lying in bed. She turns to me out of the blue and says, 'Are you all better, Mom? Are you all better?' I say, '"All better"? What do you mean, Alyssa?' 'You were mad,' she says. '"Mad"?' I said. 'Who was I mad at?' 'You were mad at Mike,' she says."

She laughed.

"It was so funny," she continued. "We were just lying there. 'Are you all better, Mom? Are you all better?...'"

As I got ready to go back to the hospital, Alyssa stood at the door and cried.

"Tell mom goodbye," she said though tears, "because she misses you."

I nodded.

"I'll do that, Alyssa," I replied.

"And I miss you, too," she added...

I spent the night on-call at the hospital. Coming home two days later, Kate greeted me, laughing.

"Mike, I have to tell you," she said. "Last night, Tommy wasn't feeling well, so he slept in bed with me while you were on call. Alyssa comes in and wants a place in the bed, and thinks Tommy is you. 'No!' she says. 'Mike, go to work!...'"

CHAPTER ELEVEN

"When I brought the children to school today, I found out that their piano teacher, Rachel, has cancer," Kate related. "She's just thirty years old. Could you imagine? Mike, what would you do if you were diagnosed with cancer?"

I took a breath.

"I'd quit the residency," I responded, "and do bioenergy with whatever time I had left."

"Mike, why don't you talk to Rachel?" Kate said. "Ask her if she'd like you to do bioenergy?..."

After the children's piano lesson I introduced myself and offered my services.

"I'd be interested in doing bioenergy," Rachel responded. "I've had experience with alternative medicine before… Allergies. Digestive difficulties. Conventional medicine hadn't helped me at all. A homeopath said my suffering was off the scale and sent me to a Chinese herbalist. I was very impressed with the homeopath for his willingness to send me elsewhere instead of using his own tools. He was incredible. He saw what needed to be done and got me in the direction of doing it. We can all do that. We're all capable of doing what we really believe in."

I hesitated.

"I'd like to do that," I responded. "Sometimes I question what I'm still doing in conventional medicine?"

"It gives you credibility," she asserted.

"But bioenergy is what I believe in most," I confided. "This is how I see myself being most useful to people. I keep asking myself, when am I going to get back to it?"

She smiled.

21

"You will," she asserted.

Rachel looked around the room.

"I'm sorry the place is so messy," she commented. "Is there any space you need to perform bioenergy?"

"No," I responded. "It doesn't matter where I am or what's going on or how I feel. Bioenergy is just what I do. It comes natural to me."

I sat across from her.

"Before we start," I said, "I'd like to try to demonstrate bioenergy to you." I held out my hand. "Guide your hand over mine and see if you don't feel anything."

She closed her eyes.

"I feel heat," she responded.

"Good," I said. "Now, let's see how far your sensitivity goes. I want you to scan up and down my forearm."

"I feel something here," she commented. "In the middle of your arm."

"Great," I affirmed. "You have a high acuity for this work. Hopefully, now you have a feeling for what I'm going to do..."

Rachel talked about coping with her condition.

"For a long time," she confided, "I've been feeling like, 'What's the point? I have this disease, and there's nothing that I can do about it.' But, now, I'm feeling better. I have a feeling that my melanoma is not going to re-occur."

She rubbed under her arm.

"Mike, I've been having a lot of pain around the site of the lymph node resection," she said. "I wonder if it could be because of severed nerves. Would you do some bioenergy on me there?"

Scanning her arm, energy radiated from the site of the excision. Following the energy's path, it quickly took me from the scar at her arm to the top of her head, then came down again in a clockwise fashion. As I circled around her, the energy flowed into the ground. Afterward, Rachel looked at me, surprised.

"The pain under my arm has disappeared," she exclaimed. "That's amazing."

"There were a couple of times that I experienced heat while you were working on me," she continued. "Had you done anything to me?"

"My work is simply a matter of following energy disturbances, and then releasing them," I responded. "Often, when blockages are removed, the normal flow of energy returns and health is restored."

She took out her purse.

"How much should I pay you?" she asked.

"No charge," I replied. "I enjoy doing this."

"Oh, but I want to give you something," she insisted.

She took a book from the shelf.

"Have you read *Jonathon Livingston Seagull?*" she asked. "You're work reminds me of the story."

I opened it to a random page and read from a passage.

Shimmering lights... Transparent... Wavered in the air...

Nodding, I looked up.

"The descriptions remind me of things I experienced while taking care of my friend, Ethel," I confided.

"Maybe you ought to write about it," she responded...

CHAPTER TWELVE

At the school carnival, an acquaintance named Jim waved me over.

"I was thinking about the bioenergy work that you do," he said. "I'm working on an electrical device called a 'bion.' It was recently approved by the FDA for the treatment of spinal cord injuries. I thought of you because it works a lot like the stuff that you're teaching at the adult school – harnessing the body's natural energy to heal."

His speech and manner radiated excitement for his work.

"I'm lacking that," I confided to Kate after Jim departed.

"Mike, you need to write a personal mission statement for yourself," she asserted...

In the evening I sat at the kitchen table, pen in hand.

Bioenergy remains the focus of my life. It treats trauma and the soul. It enlightens, and, therefore, aids everyone.

I looked in the direction of the children's room.

Residency provides security, scholarship, and funds. But when it took me too far from those I love, it had to end.

I stopped.

Why Neurology? I thought. Is it intellectual? Ego?

Washing my face I peered into my reflection in the mirror.

The light is going out, I thought...

CHAPTER THIRTEEN

"Mike, there's a friend of Rachel's here," Kate said. "Her name's Ann. She says that she's interested in bioenergy and would like to meet you..."

Ann was a self-possessed middle-aged woman.

"I had a recent fall," she said. "Since then I've had a pain in my chest."

I scanned her. A subtle energy radiated from her solar plexus. The energy held me in place for a long time.

"Most of the energy I feel is coming from your left side," I said. "Which side of your body did you fall on?"

"The left side," she said, smiling.

The energy arced to the ground. When I scanned her again, there was energy coming from her left knee. I released the strain.

"When you worked on my knee," she said, "I felt the kind of grounding energy I feel when I do Chi Gong. You can really move energy."

She sat up.

"You do have a gift," she asserted. "I think you're a lot better off following it than becoming a regular doc."

"Now, give me an argument for why I shouldn't get out of conventional medicine altogether?" I countered.

"Because you'll have the benefit of both," she answered. "There are a lot of white coats out there, but how many of them are in it to actually heal their patients? How many could recognize the bad energy in the Neurology Department at Hollywood General and make the choice that that wasn't where they wanted to be?"

"There are a lot of people who need what you can give them," she continued. "A lot more than you think."

She rose to leave.

"Well, I thank you for making this the best Sunday I've had in a long time," she said. "Whenever you start that health clinic, I'll bring the troops."

"I have connections at the community college, too," she added. "Maybe I can talk to the Dean and arrange a class for you…"

CHAPTER FOURTEEN

Paul Stanley was the Dean at Marina Community College. At the Admission Office he greeted me with a firm handshake.

"Ann told me about the kind of work that you do," he said. "I think it fits well into our self-help curriculum. If you're interested, I'd like you to teach a class..."

CHAPTER FIFTEEN

Kate pulled me aside before I left for the community college for my first class.

"Mike, I learned that one of the mothers at the children's school was just diagnosed with cancer," she said. "Her name's Angie. I told her about bioenergy and said to go to your class…"

Entering the designated classroom I surveyed the group of students inside. They ranged in age from early twenty to elderly, and appeared curious and excited to be there.

Then, my eyes were drawn to a quiet, conservative-looking woman – with dark hair and soft features – who sat in the center of the room and looked out of place there…

CHAPTER SIXTEEN

"Bioenergy is built on the concept that there's an energetic circulation to the body," I began. "One that science hasn't completely defined yet. The flow of energy within the body creates an energetic field. Trauma can lead to blockages in this field. The source of trauma can be emotional or physical, and, left untreated, manifest in disease. Bioenergy seeks to correct these blockages and restore the normal flow of energy to the body."

A woman raised her hand.

"Hi, I'm Evelyn," she said. "I want to know how exactly did you learn to do this? What was your learning curve like?"

"Several years ago I had a leg injury," I responded. "I was given medications, but all of them caused side effects: NSAIDs gave me an ulcer; muscle relaxants and benzodiazepines left me feeling like I was sleeping my life away; narcotics made me nauseous. After numerous tests and imaging studies, doctors told me I could expect chronic pain for life. In the end I came to an impasse: I could either accept things as they were, or look beyond conventional methods to alternative forms of healing. I chose the latter. That's how I found bioenergy.

"As for my 'learning curve', you might say it happened pretty quick. My first patient, I hadn't a clue. My mentor, Dr. Amin, led me into a darkened examine room where a female patient sat. She was in obvious distress. Directing her to lay on her back on the examination table, Dr. Amin moved his hand above her torso, then instructed me to do the same. 'Did you feel that?' he says. Oddly, I did – It felt like a breeze blowing against my palm. 'What is this?' I asked.
'Bioenergy,' he said under his breath. Then, he instructed me to feel for the direction the energy was moving. I felt for the energy again; it

seemed to be guiding my hand in diagonally across her torso. Dr. Amin nodded, saying the woman had been in a motor vehicle accident and suffered a seatbelt injury, and now it was our job to treat it. For the rest of the day we went from exam room to exam room, the same way."

A woman in the back motioned.

"My name's Heather," she said. "What is your take on Western Medicine and how is it different from alternative approaches?"

"My feeling is that Western approaches excel in the treatment of acute, emergent conditions," I responded, "but falls short where more chronic disturbances are concerned. Conventional medicine was born out of war. We still use terms like 'triage' and 'house officers.' It's a more aggressive approach, where something is being done to deliberately intervene. Alternative approaches are usually gentle, when the therapist works with the body to restore health."

"How does your bioenergy work?" Evelyn asked.

On the blackboard I drew a figure surrounded by energy.

"Disturbances in the energy field are found by scanning," I continued. "Moving your hand over the body till you detect energy vectors. Once you've determined the site of an energy imbalance, it can be corrected."

Evelyn sat up in her chair.

"How do you 'feel' bioenergy?" she asked.

"Let me give you a demonstration," I responded. "I call this a 'tangibility exercise.' Years ago a friend discovered that I seem to emit an energy that others are able to feel. I'm going to hold out my hand - scan it, and tell me what you find. Do you feel anything?"

She closed her eyes.

"Yes, I do," she answered. "Right there, in the center of your palm. I feel something warm."

"Good," I said. "Try moving up my arm."

She moved her hand.

"I feel something else," she said. "On your arm in the middle, but it isn't as strong as the feeling I got from your hand. Is this something you do consciously?"

"No," I replied. "It just happens. Ever since my friend discovered it, I've used it to demonstrate the technique to others."

"Can I feel bioenergy on someone else?" she asked.

"Yes," I asserted. "Would anyone like to volunteer to be scanned by Evelyn?"

Behind Evelyn was the dark haired woman with aquiline features.

"I'm Angie."

"You're Kate's friend, right?" I said. "Maybe you can volunteer for us. Evelyn, why don't you scan Angie?"

Evelyn passed her hand over Angie's body.

"I feel something here," Evelyn said. "On the right side of her stomach, but lower down. It feels round, like something in there."

"Angie, would you mind if we talked about your condition?" I inquired.

"Alright," she answered.

"Kate told me that you were diagnosed with cancer," I said. "Where is the site of the tumor?"

"It's here," she said, holding her side. "On the right, just where Evelyn said."

Gasps erupted from all four corners of the room...

CHAPTER SEVENTEEN

"Thank you," Evelyn told me at the end of class. "I was unaware of bioenergy before and how it could be used. The class definitely expanded my knowledge about the healing arts. I liked your openness and spontaneity, and your willingness to answer questions honestly. Many in the group, though, were bothered that you aren't willing to 'marry' bioenergy with your hospital work."

"Only conventional medicine is taught in a Residency program," I responded. "Anything else would be frowned on..."

Looking to the side, I noticed that Angie appeared patiently waiting and walked towards her.

"It was very intriguing," she said. "It made me want to find out more. Do you take appointments?..."

CHAPTER EIGHTEEN

Angie's home was nestled in a comfortable neighborhood of Santa Monica. Her husband, Alejandro, greeted me at the door. He was tall and soft-spoken, and seemed somewhat uncomfortable with English.

Following him into the living room, Angie was seated. She and Alejandro conversed, and I was taken by his beautiful, flowing Spanish. He then took a seat on the other side of the room.

"When I was first diagnosed with cancer six years ago," Angie began, "I was having pain on my right side. When they did an ultrasound, they found a tumor. After the surgery, they gave me chemotherapy. They said that they didn't know if the tumor would respond because I had fallopian tube cancer, and it was rare, and they didn't have a lot of experience with it.

"The chemo made me pretty sick. I didn't like it. I was fine for the next six years. Then, I went to Mexico a few weeks ago, and came back with abdominal pain and cramping. The pain was the same as I'd had six years ago. They did a CT scan, and found a mass. A biopsy showed a recurrence of the cancer. They want me to have surgery again, then go in for more chemotherapy. I don't really want to have any more chemo, and had been looking for alternative treatments. That's when Kate told me about the work that you do."

Scanning Angie energetically, a focus of energy radiated from her right side. I followed the energy till it mostly dissipated. But when I went back with the other hand, I was surprised to discover a flood of energy pouring from her navel. Tracing its path, it led me across the room to a place in the shadows where Alejandro was quietly seated.

This is a couple who share a special bond, I thought...

"I'm going in for surgery next week," Angie said as I was leaving. "Will you do some bioenergy on me while I'm in the hospital?..."

CHAPTER NINETEEN

Angie's surgery was performed at the Marina Medical Center. Visiting her in Recovery room, Angie was anxious for me to perform bioenergy.

"What do you feel, Mike?" she asked.

Scanning her, an energy vector emanated from her side. I thought it was probably because of the surgery, but its origin was further from the body than I expected, well beyond the level of the skin.

"Usually the energy from surgical incisions is close to the body," I commented. "What I'm feeling now is in the ether level… An energy layer usually related to issues of the psyche."

Continuing to scan her, it felt like there was an energy barrier surrounding her that wouldn't let me through. Tracing its outlines, it covered her like a shell from head to toe.

Then, all at once, it dissipated – like a wall coming down – and I became enveloped in a cocoon of energy and imbued with an out-of-worldly feeling.

"You have a place with these people," the feeling said...

Kate had accompanied me to the hospital. As we were preparing to leave, Angie's mother, Rosa, stopped us in the hall. She was a lovely woman with impenetrable dark eyes that were always smiling.

"Are you finished?" she asked. Her voice had a pleasant bird-like Spanish quality. "Let me pay you something. I just came from the bank, so I'm loaded."

I laughed, then turned to Kate.

"You're the business manager," I commented

"No charge, Mrs. Deuso," Kate said. "We really just came by to see how Angie was doing after the surgery…"

Walking outside to the car, I turned to Kate, perplexed.

"Why wouldn't you accept her money, Kate?" I asked. "I thought you wanted to turn this into a business?"

"There's a place for that, Mike," she responded. "Right now, I feel like being a friend…"

CHAPTER TWENTY

Angie called me following her release from the hospital. To my surprise, though, it wasn't about her.

"My sister, Petra, says that her daughter, Deanna, is always coughing," she began. "She was recently diagnosed with asthma. I told her about bioenergy and wanted to see if you could help her..."

Deanna was a child about age five. Her sullen eyes, pale complexion and frail appearance contrasted mightily with her explosive fits of hacking cough.

"It started a couple of weeks ago," Petra explained. "Just before that, Deanna had had a cold. Now it keeps getting worse."

Scanning her, a vector of energy rose from her chest. Following it I experienced a sense of child-like euphoria, immersed in feelings of wonder...

Returning to our apartment, I reviewed the literature on recent medical articles written about childhood asthma.

"Many of these articles say that symptoms of asthma start shortly after a viral infection," I told Kate. "It may be that the source of asthma isn't so much the infection as the body's response to being caught off guard. Afterwards, it seems the immune system is too hypervigilant, jumping on anything in the lung that remotely resembles an infection."

I looked up.

"What if bioenergy is able to communicate a message to the body?" I theorized. "That it's overreacting, and that overreaction is harmful? It may be that's the way we get the system to settle down."

"But don't you think that you have to do more than that?" Kate asserted. "You're just focusing on the energy part. There are other things that need to be taken care of. If the body's recovering from an infection, then it has to be replenished. There's a role for nutrition and supplements to build up the immune system. You have to instruct them on how to clean the house to get rid of anything that she's allergic to. And she needs the right medications to get her over any acute attacks…"

CHAPTER TWENTY-ONE

"Deanna's doing better," Petra told me, "but I'd like it if you worked on her again..."

Energy rose from the child's chest. It was broad and diffuse and seemed to originate a good distance from her body.

The ether level, I thought.

I followed the energy until it dissipated.

"What do you think it is, Mike?" Petra asked.

"The ether level suggests that we're dealing with emotion," I responded. "The body is overstressed."

Petra's husband, Ray, had been watching from the couch.

"So, Mike, what do other doctors think about the work you do?" he asked.

"In general, it isn't accepted," I replied.

He depressed the corners of his lips and nodded...

That evening Kate glared at me as she arrived home with the children.

"Was it so important that you go over to Petra's that you couldn't meet us at the party?" she demanded.

"Her daughter's still having problems," I responded. "You said that you wanted me to help."

"Not at the exclusion of us!" she shouted. "Goodnight. If you're not doing something at the hospital, you're off taking care of someone else."

"I'm trying to get something started, Kate," I said. "If someone benefits from the work I'm doing, maybe word will spread."

"I think it's just another excuse to be away from us," she responded, doubtful.

Well beyond her bedtime, Alyssa was frantic with exhaustion. Putting her to bed, she lay resisting sleep. Scanning her, energy radiated from her body and made a bee-line to my heart...

CHAPTER TWENTY-TWO

Angie sat in the rocking chair in her living room.

"I'm receiving daily treatments for an abscess," she said. "It developed at the site of the surgery."

Scanning over the bandage at her abdomen, a strong vector of energy radiated from the site. It had a tingly quality and emanated well beyond the skin.

"What do you feel?" she asked.

"Once again, I feel something at the ether level," I replied. "It makes me think that there's a correlation between the wound and the psyche."

She hesitated.

"I've been anxious for this thing to heal," she confided, "so that I could get on with my life."

I nodded.

"It's that feeling," I responded, "that we've been working on…"

CHAPTER TWENTY-THREE

Angie invited me to a family gathering.

"Mike, this is my Aunt Tessa," Angie said. "She's been having problems with her shoulder. Could you have a look at her?"

Scanning her shoulder, a vector of energy emanated from her scapula. Then, within an instant, the energy strain released, and she moved her shoulder up and down, then swung her arm around.

"The problem is gone," Tessa declared.

A male family member had been looking on suspiciously. Later, he pulled me aside.

"I am Angie's uncle," he said. "My name is Rico. You will have to forgive my family. Most of them are not very educated. They are superstitious and believe in magic. It is easy to take advantage of them."

Then, before I could say a word, he excused himself and walked away...

CHAPTER TWENTY-FOUR

"Dr. Yanuck, this is ER Resident, Leslie Schultz. We have an ER patient that we'd like you to admit to the floor..."

The patient's heart rate well exceeded normal limits.

"It's in the 120's," I told Schultz. "She has a history of blood clots in her lower extremities, and is complaining of worsening shortness of breath. You need to look for whether a clot has moved from her legs into her lungs."

"She's fine!" Schultz cried in a shrill voice, pacing about the emergency room as though she would pull her hair out. "She doesn't need any more of a work-up!..."

In the morning Dr. Aziz met me in the cafeteria.

"Were there any patients who you didn't admit?" he asked.

"Yeah, there was one patient in the critical care unit of the emergency room," I commented. "They called me a couple more times about her, then, suddenly, all the calls stopped."

"We better have a look at her," he responded.

In the ER the patient was missing, and Schultz stood alone in the empty space.

"The patient died," she said. "She had four children. I feel so bad..."

Standing at the door of the apartment I felt numb.

How could life be so fleeting? I wondered.

Walking through the door Alyssa greeted me, joy-filled.

"You're lucky, Mike!" she exclaimed. "You're lucky!"

"Why am I lucky, sweetheart?" I asked through the vestiges of my despair.

"Because I love you," she said...

CHAPTER TWENTY-FIVE

In the morning Alyssa woke me, excited.

"I'm a big girl now," she asserted.

Kate stood smiling behind her.

"Tell him why you're a big girl," Kate said.

"Because I made a poop in the poddy," Alyssa declared proudly. "Big poop."

Kate laughed.

"You should have seen it," Kate said. "She was so funny. She gets up, and she's looking at it, and you know how she squints her eye. 'That looks like a hot dog,' she says. 'Hot dog poo-poo...'"

In the kitchen Alyssa was playing with her dolls. Watching her I could imagine her thinking, "I can't wait to grow up."

"I've been putting that off," I thought. "Feeling unprepared and unready. Why is that?..."

At the Coronary Care Unit I sat with the nurses, exchanging stories, till I wound up telling them about my father's light-box.

"It was the only toy that I ever owned as a child," I shared. "I would spend all day pressing its buttons, trying to get all the lights to come on at once, but never could. Years later I asked my father why I wasn't able to do that - he said it was because he'd rigged it that way."

The nurses laughed.

"He set you up with an impossible task," the head nurse said...

CHAPTER TWENTY-SIX

Angie called.

"Mike, the surgical wound still won't heal," she said. "Do you have time to come over and do some bioenergy?..."

Scanning her, energy radiated from the top of her head. Following its path, it led me through larger and larger circles, till I spun like a windmill being blown by a gale-force wind. I felt uncomfortable, dancing about this way. But I had the feeling it might be doing her some good, and didn't resist it.

The energy extended higher until it got beyond my reach. For a time I was up on my tiptoes, till the energy finally came down again, flowing into my head and enveloping me in a cocoon of delightful, scintillating feelings.

Returning to where Angie was sitting, I scanned her again: Energy poured from her body, flowing like a waterfall into the ground.

"What does it mean, Mike?" she asked.

"It's a shower effect," I replied. "When a key lesion has been removed, often the other energy centers open and realign, dispelling the turbid energy that the body's been holding on to..."

Arriving home Kate and the children were seated at the table, and her oldest son, Tommy, led the prayer.

"Thank you, God, for this food, and this day, and for all of us being together," he said.

"And pray for Angie," Alyssa added...

After dinner I sat quiet on the balcony. Kate followed me.

"I don't think that there's any point to me seeing Angie anymore," I said. "I can't seem to get through. Angie always has something wall up. There's no way to know the person underneath."

"Mike, you don't know," she said. "There might be reasons for that. It might be that that's just the way she was brought up and that's the best she can do. Her family is very private."

"Some people are like that," she asserted. "They're not as open as you are. You're just going to have to get used to it. You can't hold that against them…"

The following day Angie appeared shiny and vibrant, as though a shell of frost and ice had melt away.

"I cried a lot after you left," she said. "All of the frustration over the surgery. I was finally able to let it go…"

CHAPTER TWENTY-SEVEN

At the end of a bioenergy class an older gentleman waited to talk with me.

"Hi, I'm Brian Brooks," he said. "I'm a professor at Palisades. I teach spiritual healing and have written several books on the subject."

Then, a pained expression swept his features, as he straightened and let out a sigh.

"I am also a physical sufferer of a screwed up back," he continued. "Five back surgeries, and a progressively degenerating nerve condition. I have chronic pain sometimes leading to acute pain, with increasing problems walking. I was interested in your class because I thought, somehow, what you are doing and what I am doing must connect, maybe in eternity. Who knows? Would you be willing to perform some of your bioenergy on me?"

"I'd be glad to," I said.

I directed him to a nearby chair and then began to scan him. The energy from his back seemed to have a well-defined border, like a wall. Finally, it seemed to give way, but flowed in my direction. I felt scared – apprehensive that I might be set upon by his condition – and shrank and twisted away...

CHAPTER TWENTY-EIGHT

Brian invited me to his home in Pacific Palisades. Preparing some tea for us, he moved through the kitchen with difficulty. Staring at photos attached to the side of the refrigerator, my eyes were drawn to one with an athletic-looking man crossing the finishing line at a track event.

"That was me," he commented. "Completing the Palisades Marathon."

He set a mug in front of me, then pointed to a more recent photograph in which he was surrounded by family.

"My children made a birthday party for me," he said. "I was having a good time with my grandchildren, doing the things a grandparent does – making faces – and then I noticed that I was free of all pain."

Sitting heavily opposite me, he stirred his tea.

"I think it was because I was living in my emotions," he continued. "Normally, I can't do that."

He looked at me.

"What made you decide on a career in medicine, Michael?" he asked.

"I think it was a talk I attended in high school," I responded. "A couple of oncologists from Cedars Sinai came and talked about their work with terminally-ill cancer patients. In particular, they talked about how they were using morphine to treat their patients' pain. They said they were getting a lot of flak from the medical community for doing this, because it was shortening their patients' life spans; but they were willing to put their licenses at risk if it meant easing their patients' suffering. I admired their dedication and sat there listening, thinking, 'I wanted to be a part of this fight.'"

"Where did you go to college?" he asked.

"UC Davis."

"Is that where you became interested in research?"

"That's right," I said. "During my freshman year my chemistry professor thought I had a talent for seeing things in three dimensions and took an interest in me. He taught me how to solve molecular structure with X-ray diffraction. After determining the molecular structure of a radioactive copper chelate attached to tumor specific antibodies and used to treat lymphoma, I was invited to do cancer research. I spent a year at the Weizmann Institute in Israel studying oncogenes – the genes responsible for cancer. A few years later, I was awarded a scholarship at the National Institutes of Health and developed a vaccine specifically against oncogenes to selectively kill cancer cells. It was during my work there that I suffered the leg injury that led me to bioenergy."

"What drew you to Neurology?" he asked.

"The neurological exam itself," I responded, inspired. "Examining patients with neurologic illness was like opening the hood to the human machine and being able to see how all the gears and machinery worked. Working with those patients both fascinated and horrified me at the same time: The devastation to the nervous system by neurologic disease was heartbreaking, but being able to systematically account for each and every deficit and localize them to exact sites within the brain was thrilling."

"What is the opinion of bioenergy in Neurology circles?" he inquired.

I shook my head.

"It's not accepted," I said. "While I was performing an externship at Columbia University, an article about a form of energy medicine called Therapeutic Touch was published. The study was performed by a teenage girl and concluded that the technique was ineffective. The Neurologists touted it as definitive proof that energy medicine didn't work and declaring that if there were any energetic circulation did exist, it was limited to the nervous system - entirely related to action potentials conducted through nerve cells and orchestrated by the brain."

Leaning back I remembered my time there – How oppressive it was.

"And your work suggests that it's something different?" Brian asked.

"Yes," I responded, shaking off my unpleasant thoughts. "When I perform bioenergy, I feel a certain reverence for the person I'm working on. It may be some fusion of energy between me and the other person. But I think it may come from connecting to a higher source that lay outside the brain."

He sat back.

"The brain is in charge of thinking," he said. "What you're talking about is feeling. That lay in the realm of the spirit."

He looked at me.

"Michael, do you have a faith that you believe in?"

I depressed the corners of my mouth and subtly shook my head.

"No," I responded. "I'm Jewish, but I don't really ascribe to any formal religion. I guess you could say I have no faith."

Brian lowered his gaze and leaned back in his chair.

"I've got the time of your next class marked in my calendar," he said. "I am hoping that Lucille – a client I've been treating for many years – will also be attending."

He motioned to the bookshelf.

"Mike, if you're interested, I'd like to share some of my books with you," he said. "Why don't you take a look and see if there are any of interest to you?"

I perused the titles.

"'Healers'!" I said, excited. "You wrote 'Healers'?"

I turned.

"When my mentor, Bennie Amin, taught bioenergy classes, he would read from your book," I said. "Your writings inspired me."

"Maybe I can inspire you to do some writing of your own," he responded...

CHAPTER TWENTY-NINE

Before the start of the next bioenergy class, Brian introduced me to Lucille.

"It's a pleasure to meet you," she said. "I've been suffering from dizzy spells for years."

Sitting next to Lucille was a young man with an unusually protuberant abdomen.

"I'm John," the young man. "I have an unknown form of liver disease. The doctors tell me that they're not able to diagnose it. I've tried all kinds of alternative treatments. I've even trained in forms of energy medicine before. I've tried to do something like bioenergy stuff in the past, but I think my tendency is to do it too quickly and get impatient."

Lucille was anxious to receive bioenergy and volunteered to come to the front of the class to be examined. Scanning her, I perceived an energy disturbance around her eyes.

"Would anyone else like to try to perceive the energy imbalance?" I asked.

John raised his hand and rose to scan Lucille. He looked at her intensely, then moved his hands rapidly in front of her eyes. Afterwards, he moved off and I re-examined her, and was struck by the feeling that the energy felt stuck now and locked in place, as though she'd been assaulted.

That's odd? I thought, surprised and alarmed. I've never seen anything like that happen with bioenergy before.

Looking up, John was seated now and on his face was an expression of frustration...

CHAPTER THIRTY

"Lucille came to my office feeling very sick," Brian told me. "She had a bad reaction to the work that the other person in the class, John, did with her."

I nodded, though still felt at a loss to understand.

"I could never imagine someone having a bad reaction to bioenergy," I said.

He looked at me.

"It's because John was impatient," he said. "He didn't flow with the energy – he pushed it on her."

I shook my head.

"Strange," I said. "Each time I do bioenergy, it imbues me with a feeling of reverence for the other person – Slows me down, makes me want to look deeper."

"People are different, Mike," Brian responded. "Not everyone is like you. That's why you have to be careful. Like any tool, bioenergy can be abused. If you teach it to uncaring people, it will be misused..."

CHAPTER THIRTY-ONE

Watts General lacked a Rheumatology Department, so its Residents rotated at the Palisades University Hospital for that training. On my first day of that rotation, I sat waiting for the Rheumatology attending, Dr. Blake, with a group of other Residents, who came from other outlying hospitals throughout Los Angeles and reviewed the list of Rheumatology patients admitted to the hospital.

"There doesn't seem to be a lot of work," I commented. "Only six patients on the floor – that's two patients each."

"Yeah, we're just here as cheap labor to work their public clinic," one Resident responded. "We start at noon and don't get out till nine or ten. They don't even give us a break for dinner. The rest of the time the Rheumatology attendings here are working at their private clinics – that's where they make the big bucks. They don't invite us to work there…"

Dr. Blake's secretary announced that Dr. Blake was presenting a case study in the auditorium, and told us to meet him there. Standing next to a poster, Dr. Blake explained the details of the case study.

"The patient had something called c-e-r-e-b-r-i-t-i-s," he said, enunciating each syllable. "It's a disorder of the brain."

"Yes, I'm familiar with it," I responded. "I took care of several patients with that condition when I was a Neurology Resident at Hollywood General."

He looked at me, surprised.

"Oh, you were at Hollywood?" he said, blithely. "And now you're at Watts General?… It's as though you've lived two different lives."

"There's actually a need for a Neurology Resident here," he continued. "It's a second year position that just came up because one of the Residents had to return home to Ohio for personal reasons. I'm on the Promotions Committee, so I sit in on the evaluations of all the new candidates. It might be something that you'd want to look into…"

Earlier in the week I'd told Brian about the rotation and he'd invited me for lunch at the university cafeteria. There, I told him about the interaction with Dr. Blake.

"When I said I'd been at Hollywood General, I got the feeling he didn't believe me," I confided.

I sat back.

"Maybe, I'm just being paranoid," I concluded.

"No, I understand your feelings," Brian responded. "I've worked at the University. There's a lot of snobbery and racism floating around…"

CHAPTER THIRTY-TWO

Tim Lao had been a fellow Neurology Resident during the year I spent at Hollywood General. Now, he and I were comrades in war. He was wounded, and we sat talking at the military hospital where he was rehabilitating. The Neurology staff from Hollywood General came in on rounds. They gave us a deploring look.

"This isn't some kind of reunion, is it?" Dr. Franklin said.

They walked away. Tim shook his head.

"Freedom of choice is the very cornerstone of American society," he commented...

Awakening from the dream, I showered and put on a suit. I was scheduled to interview for the posted Neurology position at Palisades today and arrived at the Department Office, briefcase in hand.

A woman approached me holding out her hand. She appeared young and energetic, though she had deep rings around her eyes.

"Hi, I'm Terry Lao," she said. "I'm a new attending here. You actually worked with my husband, Tim, while you were at Hollywood. Tim talked about you a lot. He said that of all the Residents in the Hollywood program, you had the best aptitude for Neurology, but that the program wasn't right for you. I can understand that. When Tim and I made the decision to come out here, he'd already been working in Internal Medicine for several years. When he told me that he was considering going back and specializing in Neurology, I begged him not to take the position at Hollywood. But he'd been in difficult residency programs before. He did his Internal Medicine training at Midland."

"Since he started the program at Hollywood," she continued, "he hasn't been able to spend much time with us. We moved here from Texas, and my parents are still there. My son is four years hold.

Yesterday, he was asking Tim where grandma and grandpa are. Tim explained that now that we had moved, grandma and grandpa lived in a different city. My son thinks for a minute, then turns to Tim and says, 'And where do you live, Daddy?'"

"Tim's a lovely man," I said. "I enjoyed working with him."

"You're aware that Hollywood General lost another Resident," she responded. "If you wanted to go back, I'm sure that they'd take you with open arms."

Terry flipped through my papers.

"Well, your references are outstanding," she commented. "No one has anything bad to say about you. Even Dr. Franklin, who's often critical in cases like yours, had only good things to say about you. I'm going to let our Chief Resident, Susan, take you on a tour of the department. I expect we'll be seeing you... I'm new here, but I should be a simple matter of getting your application through the Promotions Committee before you'll be able to start here..."

Susan had graduated from medical school at Hollywood.

"I didn't want to stay there for residency," she declared. "I saw what the Residents had to go through and knew it wasn't for me."

"The environment here is slow," she continued, "and the call is light. It's every fourth night, but you only admit one or two patients. How many did you usually admit at Hollywood?"

"Nine or ten," I responded.

"Yes," she said. "I guess that you were tired."

She shrugged her shoulders.

"It's just too bad Hollywood never has any luck with their choice of Residents..."

CHAPTER THIRTY-THREE

Kate phoned me at the hospital, anxious.

"The building was sold and the new owners have given me thirty-day notice to evacuate the apartment," she said. "I've been the on-site manager here for nine years, and in all that time never received even one complaint. They just want more money for the unit."

"Can we fight them?" I asked.

"No," she responded. "I've already checked with the Housing Department. They're within their rights. I have to find somewhere else for me and the children..."

CHAPTER THIRTY-FOUR

In the Rheumatology consult box was a request to evaluate a patient in the Coronary Care Unit (CCU).

"The patient has sky high blood pressure," the CCU Resident told me. "We don't know what to make of it. She has arthritis in her hands, so we thought maybe it was a rheumatology thing."

The patient had just received cardiac surgery for valve replacement. Approaching her, I was taken by the natural glow about her, and her easy manner reminded me of my beloved friend, Ethel.

"Have you had high blood pressure for very long, Ms. Ross?" I asked.

"Yes, I take medications for it," she responded, "but I've never experienced anything like this. It feels like my heart is beating into my neck."

I listened over her chest with my stethoscope and heard a significant murmur; but reviewing her progress notes, it had never been commented on.

I returned to the CCU Resident.

"The patient has a heart murmur," I said. "I hear it in all lung fields, but there's nothing documented about it in any of the notes."

"No?" he responded, defensively. "Probably an oversite..."

I called Dr. Blake and expressed my concern.

"She's followed by two attendings as well as several Residents and Interns," I said. "There's even a note from a medical student – None of them have commented on the murmur..."

"Alright," Dr. Blake said, sounding put-off. "Wait there at the Unit. I'll be there to help you when I'm done at my clinic..."

"How long are you going to be, Mike?" Kate asked. "We're waiting for you with your favorite... Potato pancakes. We have birthday cake and ice cream. I'll probably have to let the kids start eating without you…"

Dr. Blake appeared in the unit well after dark.

"Alright," he declared, bored. "Let's take a look at it."

He held his stethoscope to the patient's chest.

"There's a murmur," he said. "We'll call the Thoracic surgeon and see what he wants to do…"

We sat on a bench, waiting. Dr. Blake turned.

"I just bought some beach front property," he said. "I'd been looking at it for a long time. It finally came on the market, and I picked it up. I think that the ocean air is good for me."

I looked at the floor.

"My girlfriend has five children," I said. "The other day she was notified by the new owners of our building that she and her children had to leave."

"Oh," he responded. "That sucks."

Then, he smiled.

"How did your interviews go for the Neurology position?" he said. "I'll be interested to hear your nomination when it's forwarded to the Promotions Committee…"

The surgeon was a large man, whose treatment of the patient was mechanical and gruff.

"Sorry to call you out here," Dr. Blake said.

"Oh, that's alright," the surgeon responded. "I had to come in anyways. We've got a guy here from that hospital across the tracks with complications of another botched surgery."

Dr. Blake nudged me, smiling.

"Sounds like he's talking about your neck of the woods," he chided.

The surgeon listened with his stethoscope.

"The murmur is too loud to be meaningful," he said. "The louder they are, the less significant. It's the silent ones that are deadly."

"But it's new," I asserted.

"We'll schedule her for an echocardiogram in the morning," the surgeon responded, unhearing.

"That all sounds good," Dr. Blake asserted, merrily.

He and the surgeon discussed administrative matters and left the unit as though walking arm-in-arm…

At the apartment I ate what was left of the potato tacos. They hadn't cut the cake. Still, as I passed slices around the table, I thought that the children's faces looked sullen.

In the other room I worked on an application for a moonlighting position. Kate's older boy, Tommy, stood looking over my shoulder.

"Why does Mike need another job?" he asked.

"Finding another place for us to live is going to be expensive, Tommy," I said. "We need more money."

Tommy looked to the side, reflective.

"I want to be a doctor," he said, "who makes no money – like Mike..."

CHAPTER THIRTY-FIVE

Entering the CCU the next morning, a hush fell over the Unit. Unaccustomed to the silence, I looked about. Downcast eyes peeked up at me, then followed me disdainfully as I made my way to Ms. Ross. There, she lay in the same bed, but instead of bubbly and cheerful as she'd been the day before, she was lifeless, motionless and intubated, with a large bandage across her chest.

I turned to the CCU Resident who'd originally placed the Rheumatology consult.

"What happened?" I asked, affected.

He depressed the corners of his mouth and shrugged.

"I don't know," he said, blithely. "Her aorta spontaneously ruptured. They took her to surgery, but she hasn't woke up yet. Neurology thinks it's because her brain went without oxygen for too long – say she's brain dead."

Speechless, I knelt beside her.

The Resident looked at me, cross.

"Hey, what about that link between her high blood pressure and the arthritis in her hands?" he said. "Did you find out anything?..."

"You had it," Brian said. "You told them. I can't believe it."

He broke off.

"But I can believe that," he continued, resignedly. "That's what happens when your instructors and your peers are there for a different reason than they're supposed to – which is to help and make things right."

He shook his head.

"That's really sad," he added, solemnly. "I'm really sorry for that lady. You were there to help her – and you had the answer to help her

– and everyone blew you off..."

CHAPTER THIRTY-SIX

Along the corridors of the Palisades Hospital I walked with Dr. Blake.

"Are you ever bored at Watts General?" he asked.

"No," I said with conviction.

"What are your plans?" he asked.

"If I followed my medical calling, I'd go back to Neurology," I responded.

But these words lacked my previous conviction and struck me as insincere.

Blake turned away and other voices called to me...

"Mike, Mike," Kate called. "A letter came for you from Palisades University."

Awakening from the dream and shaking off the vestiges of sleep, I opened the letter.

"What is it, Mike?" she asked.

"It's a rejection letter from the Neurology Department," I said. "It doesn't make sense, though... They write here that they didn't fill the empty slot."

I looked at her, confused.

"It just means that they want someone else," she said...

CHAPTER THIRTY-SEVEN

Kate's brother was getting married in Nashville. Kate, the children and I flew to the wedding. As the ceremony concluded, Kate's middle son, Calvin, looked up with a knowing smile.

"Now, they get to have sex," he said with a child's enthusiasm.

"Calvin, you don't even know what sex is," his older brother, Tommy, responded.

"Yes, I do," Calvin asserted. "It's when a man gives a woman a big hug, and then an angel comes down, and blesses her, and gives the mom a baby."

Laughing, I felt my chest cave in.

"What is it, Mike?" Kate asked.

"I have this pain in my chest," I said. "I've always had it – since I was young. It started when I was at the Metropolitan museum with my uncle... He coughed, and I patted his back. Then, something happened... Suddenly, it felt like the wind had been knocked out of me. I didn't feel any pain, but I think he 'thumped' me... Hit me in the center of the chest."

"Why would he do that?" she asked.

"I don't know," I said. "Maybe it was because I bothered him."

Kate looked at me, disbelieving, and shook her head...

CHAPTER THIRTY-EIGHT

At Brian's I shared photos from the wedding. I stopped at a picture of Kate's youngest, Alyssa.

"I love her zest for life," I commented. "I love it when she starts dancing or when she shows affection for the neighbor's baby, Adrian. You can see her little mind working before those moments – You can't tell what she's contemplating until it comes out. And whenever it does, it's always in acts of joy and affection. She fills me with admiration."

"All Alyssa has to do is be her little spontaneous self," he commented.

I nodded, smiling. Then, my feeling of joy were suddenly swept away.

"Kate wants to move to Tennessee," I confided. "She thinks that the children will have a better life there."

"And what does Michael want?" Brian asked.

"I'm still held back by my fears," I said. "I'm afraid that no one will hire me after my decision to go back to Watts General."

"And what about Neurology?" he asked.

I shook my head.

"When I read my personal statement to Kate a week ago, her response was, 'You still haven't told me why you want to do Neurology.' I've been looking for the answer ever since. These days I want to understand all the workings of the body, whether it's Cardiology, Pulmonology, Hepatology, Infectious Disease…"

"And now you're in a place to do just that," he asserted.

"Still, I'm afraid," I said. "There's so much to know. What if I'm confronted with something and I don't know how to help? I don't think that I can handle that."

He rose with difficulty.

"Michael, I'm going to hold you back," he said. "You try to break free and tell me what you feel."

Brian pinned me against the wall.

"What do you feel, Michael?"

"I feel like I can't breathe," I responded.

"Why can't you breathe?"

"I don't know," I said. "It's like I've forgot how to."

He undid his hold.

"The spirit wants to be free, Michael," he said. "It's only then that you find your true self."

"You don't want to be held back, Michael," he added. "You want to let go – And you'll be fine."

He returned to his chair and sat heavily.

"I think you made the right choice in returning to Internal Medicine," he said. "Having a greater breadth of knowledge in all aspect of Medicine will profit your patients as you progress in bioenergy, which is your real calling."

Nodding, I looked through the window at the coast and thought about those times I would get off work after a thirty-six hour shift with Neurology and go to the beach and ride the waves in the water – something I hadn't done since leaving Hollywood General.

"I think it's because I felt like a prisoner there," I said, "finally freed from his cell. And I'd have to indulge that freedom by going to the beach and being close to the waves. And now that I've left Hollywood, I didn't feel that need to go to the beach. There isn't all that stress."

Then, I remembered a morning in Hollywood when I watched a patient in the Neurologic Intensive Care Unit (NICU) die in front of us.

"During the night I'd been covering for the emergency room," I said. "It was really busy that night, with lots of cases. It was standard during nights like that for the Interns to work with the upper level Resident to take care of the patients in the NICU patients. But somehow it all got away from them, and the patient didn't make it, and I couldn't help but feel that had I been there to care for the patient, it might have made the difference between life and death for him."

"And you carry that around?" Brian asked.

"Yeah," I said. "Of course. It was somebody's life. I could have made a difference."

Brian was quiet.

"You were doing the best you could," he said. "It was the system. If someone was able to save him, he was failed by the system. I don't think he was failed by the Interns, or the upper level Resident, or by you."

"And you knew it, which was why you left. You couldn't continue to abide by that."

"So leave it at the feet of the system," he concluded.

I choked up.

"But now I'm back at Watts General," I responded, "and all these programs in Neurology I'm applying to think I'm the worst Resident in the world and no one will ever give me another chance."

"But was that really what you wanted to do?" he asked. "I can't see you as a Neurologist."

"I think the decision you made was the right one," he continued. "I think you gave it more thought than you know – whether you were going to stay in Neurology or go back to Internal Medicine. I know that you feel like you made it under duress, but I think you made the right decision. Think of everything you'll be able to do. All the places that you'll be able to go to."

He leaned back.

"That day I came to your class," he said, "I knew that I was in the presence of something special. Not so much because of what you were doing for others as what I saw bioenergy doing for you. It was healing you."

"And it isn't by any accident that you're back at Watts General," he declared. "The snobs in your profession would like to make you believe otherwise, but Watts General is where you can do the most good for people – and that's important..."

CHAPTER THIRTY-NINE

"Mike, the Deuso's called," Kate said. "Angie's condition is getting worse. They're taking her back to the hospital. It looks like she needs surgery again..."

At the hospital, Angie's father, Agusto, confided their meeting with the surgeon.

"He said that the last time the tumor was around the intestines like a donut," he told me. "This time it was in sheets everywhere - on both kidneys. They tried to put in stents, but were only able to do it on one - the other kidney had to be tied off. They said that she had two months - With chemo, maybe a year. They won't be able to start treatment for five or six weeks because she needs time to heal. It will take a miracle to save her..."

Angie was wheeled to the Recovery room. She asked me to perform bioenergy and, scanning her, the energy flowed out in vortices that followed a path to my heart, as I stood, confused, unsure of its meaning?...

Returning home, I played a voice message from Brian on the answering machine.

"Mike, I'm sorry to hear about your friend," he said. "Hopefully, she'll pass away in peace and not in much pain. Take care of yourself, and remember that her soul will always be with you. She still has a lot of things that she needs you to work through for her. Listen with your heart to what her words cannot say..."

CHAPTER FORTY

After two weeks in the hospital Angie returned home. Her husband, Alejandro, arranged a party for her, complete with a band of classical guitar players.

"Mike, how are you?" he asked, greeting me at the door. "Where are Kate and the children?... Yes, tell them to come over..."

Kate and the kids arrived a short time later.

"When I told the children to put on their clothes on and get ready," she said, "the first thing Alyssa says is, 'I want to see Angie - because I can make her feel better...'"

CHAPTER FORTY-ONE

Sitting alone in the hospital cafeteria, Patel crept next to me.

"Are you tired, Mike?" he asked.

"No," I responded. "I was thinking about the night before... I've been taking care of a woman with advanced gynecologic malignancy. She doesn't have long to live. Last night, she gathered her children and told them about her illness. She'd been putting it off, worried about their feelings. Avril, her middle daughter, who seemed the one suffering with the most repressed feelings, came out of the room looking liberated - all of the children were simply glowing."

I lifted my head.

"I just wanted to hang on to the moment," I continued. "Angie's kidneys are going into failure. It's because of the expansion of the tumor. A urinary bypass procedure might buy her an extra week. I know it's not long, but if you could have just seen their faces – I just wanted the moment to go on and on."

Patel's eyes glazed over.

"Sometimes, we lose ourselves," he said, "and forget reason."

"Do you think that my thoughts are inappropriate?" I asked.

He shook his head, as though waking himself up.

"No," he said. "I was thinking about myself." He broke off. "There was an uncle who was very kind to me. He had an unusual form of cancer. It got into the bones. He died, and all I could do was ask, 'Why?'... I was there in the hospital. I had only stepped out of the room for five minutes. When I came back, he'd died."

He hesitated.

"In my religion we are taught that death is natural," he continued. "It's a normal part of life. When you die, you are born again. In medical school we learn the physiology of the body – how when the body deteriorates, it can't sustain life. But at that moment I forgot all that – asking, 'Why? Why? Why did this happen?'"

"His disease was so advanced," he added. "He didn't even have a face. Still - five minutes. Just five minutes."

"Your friend," he concluded. "You want to help her. But because of who it is, reason goes away…"

CHAPTER FORTY-TWO

Kate and Petra were organizing the candlelight vigil for Angie at the church.

"I've reconsidered on the vigil thing," Angie confided. "Things like that make me think of catastrophes like 9/11. I don't think my problem compares. It all seems a little weird to me..."

"What did you tell her, Mike?" Kate asked that evening.

"I told her that I agreed with her," I responded, "and that the first time that you told me about the idea, I'd thought it sounded a little hokey, too."

"Do you still feel that way?" she queried.

"No," I replied. "Now, I think it's a good idea – a positive way for people to express their concern."

"Did you tell her that?" she added.

"No, I didn't."

"Why not, Mike?"

"I wanted to be supportive," I said, "and validate her feelings."

"But you've got to share *all* your feelings, Mike!" she said, exasperated. "When you don't, you leave people in the dark..."

CHAPTER FORTY-THREE

In the Emergency Room a cheerful looking woman sat in a stretcher as though anchored there. I looked at the name on the chart.

"Are you 'Robert Mata'?" I inquired.

"Yes," she responded. "I know that confuses everyone. My father wanted a boy. Call me Bobbie."

"I don't know what happened," she continued. "I'd been going from doctor to doctor, telling them my legs were getting weak. Then, suddenly, they stopped working altogether."

When her reflexes were abnormal, I excused myself and went to the ER Resident.

"This patient, Ms. Mata," I said. "You have to call Neurosurgery for her at once."

"What are you talking about?" he responded. "All she has is arthritis."

"The problem isn't in her legs," I said. "It's her spine. There's something compressing the spinal cord. She needs an emergency imaging study."

Dr. Rake swooped through the emergency room.

"Yanuck, you see all these people out here!" he shouted. "It's because you keep ordering all these extra tests and getting all these crazy consults. You're jeopardizing people's lives."

He left the room, then returned with the Emergency Department Chairman.

"Dr. Rasmussen, this is that Dr. Yanuck that I've been telling you about," Rake declared.

"Oh, so you're the one who's been questioning our Emergency room attendings," said Dr. Rasmussen. "Just who do you think you are? When our attendings say a patient is ready to go up to the wards, it's your job to see that it's done. What you've committed here are atrocities, and that you were ever granted a license to practice medicine is unfortunate. I'm going to take you name, and inform the California Medical Board of your incompetence. I'll see to it that your license is revoked!..."

CHAPTER FORTY-FOUR

Holding lit candles, more than three hundred people filtered into the cathedral on the night of Angie's vigil. Kate had talked with Petra, who, in turn, spoke with Angie and got her to agree. Near the altar Angie sat in a wheelchair; the parishioners lined up and one-by-one offered prayers for her. Midway through Angie appeared weak and fading. I crept beside her.

"How are you doing, Angie?" I asked.

"I'm alright, Mike," she answered. "I thought that you couldn't be here because you're working nights at the hospital."

"I arranged coverage," I responded. "Is this becoming too much for you?"

"No," she replied. "I like it. I didn't expect so many people, though, so I'm surprised."

"I'm not," I said...

CHAPTER FORTY-FIVE

Kate and I located a home for rent near the airport. After settling on the terms, we moved in. Watching the children wander about the yard, it was like a weight had been lifted from their shoulders as they roamed in a veritable Never-Never-Land.

"After living all those years in a two-bedroom apartment," Kate said, "five of them in one room, it's like they're coming out of some long hibernation period."

Kate worked in the garden. Looking at her through the doorway, I felt blessed by the fullness of her love...

CHAPTER FORTY-SIX

Angie called and asked if I would visit?...

"Mike, I have a question," she said. "My mind isn't clear the way it usually is and it's interfering with the quality time that I want with the children. The doctors say that it could be because my renal failure is getting worse because the tumor is pressing on the kidneys. Do you think that a urinary bypass procedure will help me?"

"It might buy you a little time, Angie," I responded, "but it can also lead to problems... If the tumor spreads to the abdomen, it can result in terrible colic and pain."

She looked away.

"Then I'm back to where I started," she said...

Her husband offered me coffee in the other room.

"She had a dream last night," Alejandro said, "about being with the children. She awoke thinking that we should go on a vacation together. She likes a place on the beach in Mexico. It's about a five hour drive from here, and she wonders if she should get the kidney operation first, to make her mind more 'clear'..."

I went back to Angie's room.

"Angie, there's any number of things that could be clouding your thinking," I said. "Medicines, tumor burden, malnutrition. The renal failure is only one factor, and there's no promise that a kidney bypass will help. If you're seriously considering a trip to Mexico, I suggest you take it..."

CHAPTER FORTY-SEVEN

Angie and her family returned from Mexico.

"It was a beautiful day that Saturday in San Rafael," Agusto said. "Angie wanted to be on the beach. Rudolfo [Angie's brother] and Alejandro carried her out there. The kids played in the water. She looked really happy."

"Her blood pressure went down real low that evening, though," he continued, "and we decided that we better get her back. She was fading in and out, and I thought that they might give us some trouble at the border. But, when we got there, she woke up, and they let us through without a problem.

"Last night she gathered the family around her, and spoke to us, one by one. She said a lot of touching things - told us how good we'd been to her. It was like she was saying goodbye."

"We're having a Mass for her at 12:30," he added. "We'd like you to be there..."

At noon I returned. Agusto greeted me at the door.

"Glad you could make it," he said. "I had a question for you... It seems like Angie is short of breath. Do you know what could be doing that?"

"Well, it could be a lot of things," I responded. "Pneumonia would be the most concerning. Does she have a fever?"

Just then, Rosa crept behind me.

"Angie wants to talk to you," she said.

As I hurried to the room Rosa trailed behind me.

"She's very confused," she whispered.

Entering the room Angie's eyes appeared paralyzed, directed at the ceiling and seemingly unseeing.

"Mike, I don't want you to come anymore," she said. "I don't want people to see me like this. Don't call, either..."

Alejandro sat at the foot of the bed.

"Sorry, Mike," he whispered...

Dear Dr. Franklin,
I am writing to be considered for re-entry into the Neurology
program. Leaving was a mistake, and I hope you will accept my
apology...

CHAPTER FORTY-EIGHT

From the other room Kate called to me, and I looked up from the letter I was composing.

"Petra's on the phone, Mike," she said. "She says that Angie wants to see you…"

In Angie's room the family was gathered around her as she lay in the bed.

"Mike, I want you to do bioenergy on me," Angie said, "and tell my family how I'm going to die."

Angie could hardly move her lips now, and her voice had a piercing metallic quality.

"How long do you think I have to live, Mike?" she asked.

I knelt beside her.

"Angie, given your present condition," I said, "maybe a few days."

She hesitated.

"A few days," she said. "Well, I guess that's okay…"

I scanned her. The energy radiated up from the ether level, and made its way to my heart.

"Mike, do you mind seeing me this way?" she asked.

"No, not at all, Angie," I said. "I'm just happy to see you."

"Really, Mike?…"

CHAPTER FORTY-NINE

Dr. Guli had been my Chief Resident from Hollywood General. Now we walked side by side together along the ward.

"I needed your patient evaluations so that I can grow new," he said.

As I followed him outside, the individual stones along the walking path were inscribed with the letters for the same words – G R O W N E W...

"In the dream Guli told me all kinds of other things, too," I told Brian. "He said, 'I was trying to be kind to you,' and, 'I was trying to help you.' Yet he made my life miserable during that program, insisting that I take extra call, and making me stay late every evening."

I shook my head.

"I don't think that he was a bad person," I continued. "He was attentive whenever I presented a case – advised me, and took my calls at all hours of the night. He just didn't seem to have compassion for what I was going through."

"Did he train in an atmosphere of compassion?" Brian asked.

"Oh, no," I responded. "He trained in India. The rigors he described were frightful."

"Many times we become products of our environment," Brian commented. "It's common – though unfortunate. He was not compassionate to you because no one had shown him compassion."

Then, he closed his eyes, and leaned back.

"What was your first impression of Hollywood's Neurology Department when you interviewed there?" he asked.

"I thought that I could hide there," I responded. "Complete my residency, and then quietly go back to bioenergy. The moment that I met the Chairman, Dr. Franklin, he struck me as oddly detached and unconnected. When he spoke, I never had the feeling like there was someone else in the room with me. It was as though he had no physical presence."

"He was all in his head," Brian interjected. "He was all thinking and no feeling."

"He seemed like a good man," I said. "He was a good teacher. He preached high principles. The problem was, when I needed him to fight for me, he couldn't – or wouldn't."

"As the Chairman of the Department he formed the nucleus for the people who he brought in," Brian responded. "It was no accident that his staff was so unfeeling. Your Dr. Arnold, who treated you so cruelly, had no warmth. It was no accident that he worked for Dr. Franklin. The same can be said for your 'friend' and Chief Resident, Dr. Guli."

"But, in the end, he was a friend to you," he continued, "and he did help you, as did all of the Neurologists at Hollywood General. They gave you a skill that will serve you for a lifetime. They showed you how a medical center should run, and helped send you to a place where your help was desperately needed. This might not have happened at another Neurology program. At someplace else, you probably would have 'slid by', as seemed your intention. They helped you realize the importance of kindness in training others, so that you can remember that when one day you're in a position of training medical students and Residents."

Depressing my lips, I shook my head.

"I'll never be in that place," I lamented. "I've ruined my career."

He looked at me.

"Michael, you represent change," he declared. "You want a world of kindness, compassion and understanding, and are willing to fight for it – take risks for it. The change will come."

He moved forward.

"You've been through a kind of purgatory," he said. "You've been purged. Now, do what the dream said… 'Grow new.' That's the message.

"And you are a man of faith, Michael. You believe in a healing power, even though you can neither see nor measure its effect."

"And I believe, too," he concluded, "because I've seen you heal with bioenergy – and I've seen it heal you…"

To: Eugene Rasmussen, M.D.
Chairman, Department of Emergency Medicine

From: Thomas Shigura, M.D.
Chairman, Department of Internal Medicine

This letter concerns my Senior Resident, Dr. Michael Yanuck, for whom you threatened to report to the Medical Board. I also met with Dr. Abbassi Aziz, who was present at the time you made that statement and corroborates your comments.

The flurry of e-mails you send me almost daily about 'inappropriate' admissions to various units by Dr. Yanuck follows this pattern of behavior. As you recall, I have had each case investigated and determined that none of the cases you mentioned were inappropriately managed, nor admitted to the incorrect unit.

I believe your conduct and behavior are inappropriate and clearly unprofessional. You have harassed my Residents and this is a violation of hospital policy. I am copying this memorandum to the Disciplinary Action Hearing Board, and they will have to handle it.

I am disappointed that you have had to resort to such conduct...

CHAPTER FIFTY

Patel approached as I entered the hallway.

"Dr. Yanuck, the patient you saw in the emergency room who wasn't able to use her legs, Ms. Mata, would like to talk to you," he said. "Neurosurgery was called the way that you instructed, but, by the time they got to her, it was already too late. An MRI showed a tumor in her spine. The source turned out to be colon cancer. Oncology was consulted. They say that her condition is terminal and there isn't much they can do…"

Ms. Mata sat in the bed, looking much the way she did when I first met her.

"I have difficult news, Ms. Mata," I said.

"Call me Bobbie," she said. "All of my friends do."

I sat next to her.

"Bobbie, you have cancer," I said.

Her eyes drifted, and a stillness seemed to creep over her.

"How long have I got left?" she asked.

"We can't know for sure," I said. "We're working with the cancer doctors, and we'll do all that we can. But considering the advanced stage of the disease, it might be only months."

"Have you taken care of patients like me before?" she inquired.

"Yes, Bobbie," I responded. "Not long ago I took care of a friend with pancreatic cancer. I'm writing a book about her."

"Have you finished your book?" she asked. "If you have a copy, I'd like to read it…"

CHAPTER FIFTY-ONE

Petra called from Angie's.

"The family is worried about Alejandro," she said. "Angie hasn't slept in the past twenty-four hours, and he still insists on taking care of her by himself..."

At the house Angie tossed in bed, unable to find calm.

"I don't care if it means ten years out of my life," Alejandro said. "I'm going to take care of her."

Angie's mother and father left the room. Agusto appeared exhausted and paced the floor.

"Why?" he repeated. "Why, God? Why?"

Rosa's face was flushed. Her ears ringing, she began to weep.

"Would you like to get some air outside, Rosa?" I asked.

She sat on the patio. In the moonlight I scanned her. The energy that emanated from her had a scintillating quality - like a swarm of fire-flies, flashing one by one, before disappearing into the night.

"You will go to heaven," she said, "because you are a beautiful person..."

Returning to the room, I asked Alejandro if I could work with Angie? He nodded, and stepped back. Scanning Angie, I was immediately gripped by feelings of delight. Soon, she was resting comfortably and told her family goodnight.

Alejandro turned to me.

"Would you like something to drink, Mike?" he said.

He prepared some coffee, then sat with me at the kitchen table. I looked at him, smiling.

"I always enjoy doing bioenergy with Angie," I said. "She has such a wonderful spirit."

Nodding, his eyes glazed over.

Then, he laid his head on the table and wept...

CHAPTER FIFTY-TWO

Awakening in the morning the word 'Love' sprang into my head. Rolling over Alyssa lay asleep next to me.

"Hello, beautiful one," I said.

Smiling, her face radiated with delight. I bent low and kissed her forehead.

"I'll see you a little later."

She turned, still smiling...

Outside, I took Tommy and Calvin for a bike ride, up-and-down the hills near the house.

"Come on, boys," I said. "It's time to get back. Your father will be here soon."

"One more hill," Tommy insisted...

The children's father, Tomas, was waiting at the house when we returned. He packed the children in the van and took them to their grandmother's. I turned to Kate and suggested we take a walk.

"Maybe, you'd like to talk," I said.

"What about?" she asked.

"About us."

"Not particularly," she responded.

She said that I'd never made any presupposes about wanting to have a family. I had always been clear.

"We'll live as roommates," she said. "After that, I'll get a job or go home to Tennessee..."

She said that she had to go to Ikea. I asked if she'd like me to come with her?

"It didn't matter," she responded.

At the checkout counter I went to pay for her things.

"You don't have to."

We got in line for Swedish meatballs. I felt happy and asked for a friendly kiss...

CHAPTER FIFTY-THREE

In the afternoon Tomas returned with the children. Kate rented a video, and she and the children sat watching it in the living room, while I stayed locked in the bathroom, hunkered over my books – the sounds of their laughter creeping in through the keyhole.

Later, I called to check on Angie. Petra answered the phone.

"Hi Mike," she said. "We're watching a movie... *Big Fat Liar...*"

"Oh, I've heard of that," I said, absently.

It was the movie Kate and the children had been watching...

CHAPTER FIFTY-FOUR

Brian laughed as I shared the *Big Fat Liar* coincidence.

"Michael," he said, "one of my favorite quotes comes from Henri Nouwen – 'The Heart is more important than the head - Being is more important than doing - Doing things together is more important than doing things alone.'"

He poured tea and sat heavily beside me. Then, he pointed to a jar on the bookshelf.

"You see that over there?" he said. "Bring it to the table."

The jar was heavy. Inside was a metal contraption that looked like a giant, sinister, mechanical spider.

"That came out of my back," he explained. "When they had to re-do my spinal fusion surgery a few years ago, I asked if I could keep it."

Viewing the device it seemed to resemble an iron claw.

Like an instrument of torture, I thought.

"The second fusion didn't go much better," he continued. "My health keeps taking interesting side trips. The neurologist now is convinced that I not only have a bad back and degenerating nerve condition, but also restless leg syndrome. This accounts for my problems at night and not sleeping."

I nodded.

"You'd think that I'd feel at home with neurological conditions like yours," I commented. "After all, it was only a year ago that I was training at Hollywood General to become a Neurologist."

"Disorders of the nervous system frighten you," he responded. "You chose Neurology to specialize in because you were looking to overcome your fears and come face-to-face with them."

"I don't think there's anything that scares you as much as conditions of the nervous system," he continued. "You like to be in control. It's natural."

I looked into the jar again, then put it back on the shelf.

Brian leaned back.

"I saw the orthopedic doctor yesterday," he said. "He read both my MRI and X rays, and concluded that both shoulders are shot and need replacements. He said my shoulders are bone on bone, and have arthritic spurs. He was a very young guy, and said it was really my call on how much pain I can take and a lifestyle issue. He did give me a cortisone shot, and scheduled me to get some special therapy sessions."

He attempted to rotate his shoulder.

"I think that I know all the exercises, but I am willing to learn more," he added. "The shot I think has helped, but it is a little early to tell."

I began to scan him energetically, then stopped, feeling overwhelmed.

Oh, what am I doing? I thought. This is serious stuff that he's dealing with, and I'm here waving my hands around – practicing some healing art with no credentials.

"In the origins of faith," Brian said, "there was never a single founder who came forth with any credentials."

He looked at me.

"Michael, God is love," he said. "I believe that love is a part of the work that you're doing. You have a gift. Despite considering myself a skeptic, I have faith in you."

I scanned him again. His energy merged with my own and in that moment I had the feeling of being at one with everything around me, as time slowed, and nothing else seemed to matter.

"I can feel the vertebrae between my spine opening," Brian declared. "I hear it – pop, pop, pop – up and down my back."

He stood, rotated his hips from side-to-side and swung his arms back-and-forth.

"I haven't been able to do that in years," he said. "I can't remember the last time I've had this much mobility."

In my body the energy encircled me, then flowed upward.

"What are you feeling, Michael?" he asked.

"I feel – reverence," I answered. "The answer – to follow it, work with it, take it where it needs to go – I've always known."

"But now you understand," he said...

CHAPTER FIFTY-FIVE

Leaving Brian's, my body bristled with energy – teaming with it as never before. At home Alyssa met me at the doorway.

"Mike, come and play," she said.

Slowly, the energy began to dissipate. Then, suddenly, I experienced a sensation like a shift in my spine.

"Ahhh," I emitted.

"Ah-woo!" she sang.

She thinks I'm playing, I reasoned. Like the vocalizing we usually do for fun.

Just then, another 'shift' ripped through my back and brought me to my knees.

"Whoa," I said.

"Whoo-wee!" she cried.

I laughed, and she giggled with me. As I knelt on all fours laboring to get to my feet, Alyssa danced around me: It were as though I were at the center of some Native American ceremony.

Finally, I got up, and found that I was standing straighter and taller than before, and breathing with greater ease.

"Whew," I said.

"Whew-ah," responded Alyssa, and ran an exhausted arm across her forehead, so to remove the sweat from her brow...

Mike,
Your 'book' is a document to self-indulgence that is filled with
delusions, deceptions and inaccuracies. It is rather pathetic...
William Brand...

CHAPTER FIFTY-SIX

As I sat re-reading Dr. Brand's letter, the phone rang. I was so consumed with heartache that I didn't even look up.

Kate answered it. From the tone of the conversation, I presumed she was talking with an old and dear friend.

"Yes, yes," she said. "It's nice to talk to you, too… Yes, Mike has told me so much about you. Here he is."

Then, she came into the room and handed me the receiver.

"Mike, it's for you," she insisted. "It's your patient… Bobbie…"

"I just finished reading your book," Bobbie exclaimed in excited tones, "and I had to call you immediately to tell you to stop procrastinating and publish it!"

No, I said. I would never publish it. It would never see the light of day. I had just received a letter from my former instructor. He had cared for Ethel with me and disapproved of the book, even accusing me of lying. There was nothing to do but shelve it.

"You write your truth, Michael!" she insisted. "Some people are like that. They feel like they have a lot to protect. Don't let that stop you. Put it in print!…"

Arriving on the ward the following morning I was looking forward to seeing Bobbie. But entering her room, I found the bed was stripped and dressers empty.

"She died during the night," Patel explained. "Her heart rate slowed, and then her vitals faded. When we got to her, she was already gone…"

"I can't believe it!" Kate exclaimed. "She was so alive on the phone. 'Kate? – Is this Kate?' she said. 'You sound just like Mike described you when he was telling me about you.' She talked to me just like we'd been old friends. It just goes to show you how fragile life is."

"You must have made quite an impression on her, Mike," she continued. "She said that she'd been married, but that she'd never had a child, and that you were the closest thing that she ever had to one – like you were her own son..."

CHAPTER FIFTY-SEVEN

"You couldn't save her, Michael," Brian said. "I know how much you wanted to, because you want to save everyone, but it was her time."

I lowered my head.

"I wish I'd had the opportunity to do bioenergy with her," I responded.

He leaned back in his armchair.

"When I studied Asian spiritual practices," he began. "I went to Beijing where I observed Chi Gong Masters teaching medical students at the Beijing Hospital. I went with them all over the hospital and watched them take care of every kind of patient – Except cancer patients – I didn't see them work with cancer.

"So I asked one day if they worked with cancer? And they said they didn't like to do that, because too many of their students had died of basically absorbing the cancer from the patients and then getting the malignancy themselves.

"They said the danger was, if you don't clear the pathogens of patients properly or enough, they start compounding. So you need to be strong enough in your connection to heaven & earth, the body-mind or whatever word you want to use to actually know how to work with cancer, and it could take years and years to cultivate.

"And I think it's important to understand this, because I know you work with people with cancer, and if you work with cancer..."

He broke off.

"The Masters told me," he resumed, "for someone to be good at working with cancer, they have to be so clear in themselves and their connection to the heaven & earth and the divine energy - And impeccable in your energy work and purification work, so that you don't leave residual energies behind that can slowly accumulate toxins in the body and then create other manifestations of disharmony within you which can be detrimental.

"So if you have concerns that you're not safe, you shouldn't be doing the work. And it's unfortunate, but you have to ask yourself that question."

I looked at him. It was true I'd been afraid of contracting neurologic illness – like I'd been with him till he got me over that fear. But I had no such fear with cancer; I saw cancer as mainly a breakdown in communication between single cells and the body as a whole: Each cell is there to promote the general welfare of the person; each has self-suicide pathways for when things go wrong. In response to being exposed to carcinogenic toxins and mutation-causing free radicals, the cell turns on these self-suicide programs, so to self-destruct and thereby protect the organism as a whole.

It's only when the genes for these self-suicide pathways get mutated that these cells become malignant – because then those self-destruct mechanisms can't be turned on. That's when malignant transformation occurs.

But, even then, I'd seen in the test-tube that there were ways of triggering what was left of the cell's self-suicide pathways. And I'd developed a vaccine that activated the immune system to attack cancer cells. And this was what I hoped bioenergy was able to tap into when helping a patient with cancer.

Brian nodded.

"You're not incorrect," he responded. "Mostly, the Chi Gong Masters talked about how they had to get the immortal aspect to go dormant, so that the cancer can turn back into a regular cell, so it can slough off and the mass shrink and go from solid to liquid and disperses.

"So you're correct. That's how they worked with the mass. They worked with the underlying emotional roots. The goal was to get that shift of perspective from the original insult."

I looked away. I hated the thought of cancer having an 'emotional' basis – It was just too hurtful – Like blaming the person because they weren't able to manage their feelings and, in that way, brought the cancer on themselves!

"I prefer to think of cancer as caused by problems like smoking," I said, "and the harm that does to cells until you get to one that becomes cancerous."

"But, whatever the cause," I continued, "I wonder that bioenergy could still effect a communication with the cancer cell? Say, 'The person's sorry for what he or she has done in the past and won't do it again. Now it's time to activate what's left of your self-destruct mechanisms, so the body can heal and the person's health be restored.'"

"You're right in what you said," Brian asserted. "That dialogue… The Chi Gong Masters didn't use those words, but what you're saying is correct in its process.

"It's just that when you're talking about cancer and telling cancer cells to lay down their lives for the general good, it's like asking a contentious five-year old to give up his favorite toy because that's the better thing to do – And that doesn't always go well."

I nodded, grimly.

No, it hadn't gone well, I thought. When I cared for Ethel, my work might have helped with her transition from this world to the next, but I didn't think that it had helped her when it came to the growth of the cancer. I recalled viewing those follow-up imaging studies: Despite having worked with her with bioenergy, the growth of the cancer was stunning, so to leave me feeling wholly impotent. And now Bobbie was dead. And Angie didn't have much time.

"Mike, when I was in Beijing… Well, in those days, I could be pretty cocky… I asked, 'Who's the best doctor? I want to learn from him.' They pointed me to this one Master. I went over and started talking with him and asked what his success rate was? How many people he healed? What percentage? He said, '100%.' I said, 'You heal them all?' He said, 'Yeah, I heal every single one of them. But they don't all live.'"

Brian chuckled and I couldn't help but joined him.

"But in time I realized that much of their work involved things like helping the spirit exit the body, gathering up all the energy the person had left, so that it's easier for the soul to transition in a clean fashion.

"And then there is what they called, 'Forgiveness work', that releases the emotional ties – the karmic ties – between the patient and everyone that they've ever met. And when they got to that point, it created tremendous healing – for their spouse, for their offspring, for their parents. Because when final forgiveness is finally granted, what you have is a place of gratitude for the experience that took place, so that you're ready to leave this place of pain."

My mind drifted to Ethel: In those last hours I felt like I'd betrayed her by not recognizing how close she was to death; what she was trying to tell me in her paralyzed state when she couldn't speak or move her limbs; I didn't get her to the emergency room like she probably wanted; I'd failed her that way.

Nevertheless, she'd let me wipe away her tears in those final moments – and later her soul came to comfort me when I understood what happened and I was overwhelmed with guilt.

"You've taken this discernment into a place of gratitude," Brian continued.

Nodding, I considered my conversation with Bobby: It was as though, in her last words, the most important thing was for her to support me.

"You speak your truth…"

CHAPTER FIFTY-EIGHT

Angie's brother-in-law, Ray, managed the Trader Joe's near the house. He was standing at the checkout counter when I entered the store.

"Angie went to see *Harry Potter* today," he said. "She keeps hangin' in there. She looks thin, but her mind's sharp. She drinks a lot of juice. I think she wants to stay around for a while. Her family takes good care of her, too…"

Later in the morning a call came from the hospital.

"Dr. Yanuck, we have some perspective Interns for the program," the Department secretary said. "Would you mind giving them a tour?…"

"Why did you choose Watts General to do your internship?" an applicant asked.

"The decision was mostly personal," I responded. "In medical school most of my patients were African American. Then, just before I finished, a close friend died. I wanted to come home to California. I interviewed at Watts General, and everything just seemed to fall into place."

I looked away.

He probably thinks I'm full of it, I thought.

He stood smiling, nodding his head.

"You wanted to give back," he said. "I admire you…"

Kate met me at the door, smiling.

"Calvin and Sandra were fighting today," she said. "Alyssa gets that serious look on her face - she says, 'Sandra. Calvin. No fight.

Friends.' Then she goes and gives Calvin a hug. Then Sandra. 'Friends,' she says."

"Later, Sandra wasn't behaving," she continued, "so I swatted her on the butt. Alyssa got very upset. 'Why you hit Sandra? No hit Sandra.' And she gets that serious look and starts bopping back-and-forth and talking to herself. She was very pained..."

Kate and the children sang in bed.

"Sing, Momma," Alyssa said. "Sing, guys," she said to the other children...

"I swear, Mike," Kate said, laughing. "All your picture taking, and Alyssa's the picture taking pro now. 'Come on, guys,' she says. 'Take picture. Okay. 'Nother one...'"

In the afternoon I visited Angie. As I performed bioenergy with her, I confided Kate's concerns about Alyssa and my overindulgence.

"I can't seem to help myself, though," I said. "I love to watch her. For me she can do no wrong."

Having taken the energy through its path, I sat beside Angie.

"Kate says that I spoil Alyssa," I continued. "I probably do."

"She really loves you," Angie commented.

And looking into her eyes they looked more radiant and alive than I'd ever seen them...

CHAPTER FIFTY-NINE

Ray called.

"Earlier in the morning Angie expired," he said. "Petra and the family were wondering if you'd give the eulogy at the funeral..."

At the Cathedral the school children filed into the sanctuary; their parents sitting along the aisles. From the pulpit I looked out.

"Angie touched us with her courage," I said. "In a dream she saw herself making time for her children on the beaches of San Felipe – Then, made it a reality. She cared for those around her – When the time of her passing grew nearer, she prepared them.

"And in her final days, what was she doing? When I called, it was, 'Mike, we'll have to get back to you. We're going on a stroll', or 'Mike, Angie's not here. She went to see *Harry Potter*.. Or 'Mike, we're on our way to the beach. We'll call back.'

"Angie and her family let us into their lives that we may learn from their example. Her husband, Alejandro, and his unwavering devotion; her parents, Agusto and Rosa, and their unfailing care; her brother, Rudolfo, and sister, Petra, and their unfaltering vigilance.

"We, as a congregation, have been blessed..."

At the cemetery Alejandro stood at the head of the family, and acknowledged well-wishers as they passed Angie's coffin. When I arrived at the front of the line, Alejandro embraced me.

"Thank you, Mike," he said, "for all you done. When you called it gave me energy, even when I couldn't go on."

"You were always there for us," he continued. "It helped a lot. You got me through difficult times. I always knew I could call you. I knew you were out there. Thank you. Thank you, Mike..."

Kate crept behind me.

"Alyssa overheard me talking about Angie," she said. "'We need to take her to the hospital,' Alyssa says. 'Well, she's already dead,' I told her. 'Well, maybe they can make her better,' she said. 'No, honey,' I said, 'God's taken her to Heaven.' Then she puts her head down. 'I really miss Angie,' she says, and sheds a tear…"

At the reception a man sitting with an older woman waved me over.

"My mother heard your eulogy," he said. "She wanted to know how you are related to Angie."

"I'm a doctor," I said. "I helped take care of her during her final months."

The son translated for her. She nodded, and then looked at me.

"I don't know how to say this because I speak in Spanish, and I don't know English good," she said. "When the children growing up, we all live close. Rosa in the house next to me. I see her all the time with the kids. Rudolfo had his arms around his mother like this – Holding tight to his mother's leg. I want Rosa to have a rest, so I say, 'Rudolfo, you come to my house.' He pulls tighter at Rosa. 'No, no,' he says. Then, little Angie takes my hand. 'I go with you,' she says.

"During the night before I come here, I feel nervous – crying – all night – no able to stop. Then I feel someone take my hand. It was Angie. Just like when she small. I could see her upper half, but legs were blurry - I can't see her feet. 'I go with you,' she says. Just like that.

"I don't say this to nobody. They think I'm crazy. Some things impossible to explain. I think she not in Heaven yet. I think she still here – Make sure everyone okay…"

Driving home I was mostly silent.

"What are you thinking, Mike?" Kate asked.

I kept my eyes fixed on the road ahead.

"It's a funny feeling I'm left with," I responded. "One of service…"

ABOUT THE AUTHOR

Michael Yanuck MD PhD is a physician-scientist
whose groundbreaking research at the National Institutes of
Health was the basis for a FDA-approved vaccine for cancer.
Following a traumatic leg injury he returned to Medicine. Intent
on helping those most in need, he enlisted in the National Health
Service Corps, worked in urban and rural health centers throughout
the country, then served native peoples with the Indian Health
Service. Currently, he cares for homeless Veterans and serves as
Pain Care Champion for the Northern California VA.
He continues to practice bioenergy, which
he teaches to the public.